Menopause for Men

Jennifer Erchul

ISBN: 9798300340964

DEDICATION

To Rory, my brave and bewildered partner in this hot adventure—

Your frustration, confusion, and complete lack of menopause knowledge inspired me to write this book. Hopefully it helps other women through the journey…because their man gains some more knowledge in their hormonal hell.

Here's to surviving the storms, celebrating the calm, and finding humor in the hormonal hurricane.

With love and laughter,
Jennifer

CONTENTS

Extras:

Introduction: Welcome to the Menopause Show!

Picture this: You're sitting in the comfort of your living room when, out of nowhere, your usually composed partner suddenly bursts into tears over a commercial. Ten minutes later, she's furiously adjusting the thermostat, mumbling something about the house being a furnace. Then, as if flipping a switch, she's laughing uncontrollably at a joke you didn't even finish. Congratulations—you've entered the menopause zone!

Menopause might not be something you expected to deal with (hey, you didn't sign up for hormonal chaos, did you?), but here you are. And here's the good news: you're not alone, and you can survive this. In fact, with the right mindset, you might even come out of it a stronger, more empathetic partner.

This book isn't about turning you into a doctor or hormone expert—it's about giving you the tools to navigate this new chapter in your relationship. From practical tips to understanding the science behind the hot flashes, we've got your back. You're in for a ride, but with humor and heart, we'll help you buckle up and hang on.

ACKNOWLEDGMENTS

To all the incredible women who've weathered the hot flashes, mood swings, and sleepless nights with grace (or at least wine)—this book is for you.

Thank you to the warriors who shared their menopause stories, from the hilariously unfiltered to the deeply insightful. Your candor about sweating through board meetings, crying over cereal commercials, and arguing with thermostats is what inspired me to put pen to paper.

To those who took the time to educate the men in their lives—patiently explaining that "no, I'm not mad at you, I'm mad at everything"— thank you for paving the way. The world is a better place when the menfolk know the difference between empathy and "just calm down."

And to every woman who passed down survival tips like they were the sacred wisdom of our foremothers—whether it was about layering clothes like a pro or finding the perfect chocolate stash hiding spot— you are the real MVPs.

Ladies, we've survived this rollercoaster with humor, heart, and probably a little too much caffeine. Thank you for reminding me (and everyone else) that even in the madness, there's sisterhood.

With gratitude, laughter, and maybe a few cooling patches,
Jennifer

1 THE HORMONAL ROLLERCOASTER

Let's start with the basics: hormones. Think of these as the tiny chemical messengers that control everything from her mood to her metabolism. In her 20s and 30s, her hormones were like a well-rehearsed symphony—beautifully balanced and harmonious. Then, somewhere around her 40s, the conductor (estrogen) decides to retire, leaving the orchestra in chaos. Welcome to the hormonal rollercoaster.

The Science (Simplified for You, the Non-Physician)

There are three key players in this hormonal drama:
- Estrogen: The star of the show. Keeps everything running smoothly, from her skin to her sanity.
- Progesterone: The peacekeeper. Helps balance out estrogen and keeps things calm.
- Testosterone: Yes, women have it too, and it's what gives her energy and libido a boost.

During menopause, estrogen starts packing its bags, progesterone quietly exits stage left, and testosterone hangs around just enough to keep things interesting. The result? Chaos.

The Symptoms: AKA, What You're About to Witness

1. Hot Flashes: These aren't just "feeling a little warm." Imagine her inner thermostat breaking and deciding it's time to roast marshmallows—inside her body.

o Pro Tip: Keep a fan nearby and resist the urge to cuddle her mid-flash.

2. Mood Swings: One minute, she's laughing at a dog video. The next, she's crying because the dog is too cute. The hormones are to blame, not you (probably).
o Pro Tip: Validate her feelings, even if you don't understand them.

3. Brain Fog: Ever heard her ask, "What was I doing again?" That's menopause messing with her memory.
o Pro Tip: Gently remind her without teasing—unless she's in the mood to laugh about it.

4. Sleeplessness: If she's tossing and turning all night, you're not sleeping either. Insomnia is a common side effect of fluctuating hormones.
o Pro Tip: Offer to adjust the thermostat or grab her a glass of water. Small gestures go a long way.

Your Role in the Rollercoaster Ride
Think of yourself as the guy operating the safety harness. You can't stop the ride, but you can make it safer and more bearable for both of you. This means:
• Being Patient: Yes, it's hard when she's short-tempered or emotional, but she's not doing it on purpose.
• Being Observant: Notice what triggers her symptoms (heat, stress, spicy food) and help mitigate them.
• Being Proactive: Learn her new needs—whether it's cooling pajamas or a stockpile of snacks—and meet them without being asked.
The Humor in Hormones
It's okay to laugh about it. In fact, laughter might be your best weapon. When she's fanning herself with a magazine and yelling at the dog for breathing too loudly, find the humor—not at her expense, but in the absurdity of it all.

This sets the stage for deeper dives into specific symptoms, emotional impacts, and how men can be active participants in navigating menopause with grace—and a good sense of humor.

2 MENTAL AND EMOTIONAL WHIPLASH

If you've noticed that your partner's emotions have started resembling a hurricane—calm one moment, raging the next—you're not imagining things. Menopause is the culprit, turning her usually stable mental and emotional state into a wild ride of highs and lows. Here's the thing: it's not personal. It's biological. And understanding this can make all the difference.

What's Happening Inside Her Brain?

Hormones like estrogen don't just affect the body; they play a critical role in regulating the brain. When these hormone levels fluctuate, they can wreak havoc on emotions, mood, and even cognitive functions. In simple terms, her brain chemistry is playing a new and unpredictable tune.

- Estrogen and Mood: Estrogen helps regulate serotonin, the brain's "feel-good" chemical. When estrogen dips, serotonin takes a hit, leading to irritability, sadness, or anxiety.
- Cortisol Chaos: Menopause can also heighten stress hormone levels, making her more sensitive to everyday frustrations.
- Brain Fog Alert: Forgetfulness and trouble concentrating aren't intentional—they're a byproduct of hormonal shifts.

How This Feels for Her (and Looks to You)

Picture this: She's crying over a commercial about kittens one moment and furious because you didn't load the dishwasher "correctly" the next. This emotional whiplash can feel confusing for her—and downright baffling for you.

But here's a secret: she's likely just as surprised by these emotional surges as you are. Imagine your feelings getting hijacked without warning. It's unsettling, and it's not her fault.

What You Can Do (Without Getting Hit by a Flying Shoe)

1. Validate, Don't Minimize: When she's upset, avoid phrases like "You're overreacting" or "Is this menopause?" Instead, say something like, "That sounds frustrating. How can I help?"
2. Be Present: Sometimes, she doesn't need a solution—just a listening ear. Put down your phone, make eye contact, and let her vent. Bonus points if you nod sympathetically.
3. Pick Your Battles: If she's arguing about something trivial, ask yourself: "Does this really matter?" Most of the time, it doesn't.

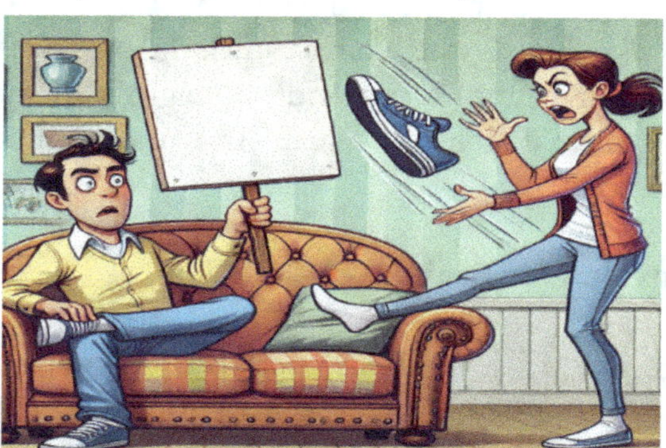

Let it slide.

4. Plan for the Unexpected: Keep snacks on hand. Blood sugar dips can make emotional swings worse. A strategically offered chocolate bar can be a lifesaver.

The Humor Factor

Navigating mood
swings can feel like walking through a minefield,
but humor is your secret weapon. Lighthearted moments can help defuse tension:

•   Example: If she's ranting about how the dog is staring at her, respond with, "He's just wondering how you manage to look so fabulous even when you're mad." (Note: Only attempt this if she's
in
a slightly good mood.)

Pro Tips for Emotional Support

•   The Three Magic Words: Not "I love you" (although those are great, too), but "I've got this." Whether it's taking over chores or picking up takeout, show her you're stepping up.

•   The Power of Quiet Gestures: Surprise her with her favorite tea or draw her a bath without being asked. These small actions say, "I see you, and I care."

Quick Cheat Sheet: What Not to Do
•   Don't Play the Hormone Card: Even if her mood seems hormone-fueled, calling it out is like throwing a lit match into a gas tank.
•   Don't Take It Personally: If she snaps at you, remember it's likely not about you—it's about the physiological chaos she's dealing with.
•   Don't "Fix" Everything: Sometimes, she just wants to be heard, not helped.

Why This Matters
Emotional support during menopause isn't just about surviving her mood swings—it's about strengthening your connection. Showing her you're willing to understand and adapt builds trust and intimacy during a   challenging   time.

3 PHYSICAL CHANGES

Menopause doesn't just impact a woman's emotions and mental state—it also brings a parade of physical changes that can be both perplexing and, let's face it, frustrating. As her body adjusts to fluctuating hormones, you may notice shifts in everything from her energy levels to her waistline. Here's your crash course on what's happening and how to be her supportive partner through it all.

The Hormonal Domino Effect on Her Body

1.   Weight Redistribution:
o   What's Happening: Hormonal shifts can lead to weight gain, particularly around the midsection. Think of it as her body's misguided attempt at self-preservation.

- Your Role: Avoid the dreaded "Are you eating more?" question.
  Instead, support her in maintaining a healthy lifestyle by offering to join her on walks or trying new recipes together.

2.   Skin and Hair Changes:
o   What's Happening: Lower estrogen can result in drier skin, thinning hair, and a newfound appreciation for moisturizer.

- Your Role: Compliment her often. Her confidence might take a hit, but your kind words can make a big difference.

3.   Bone Density Loss:
o   What's Happening: Menopause increases the risk of

osteoporosis, which means her bones need extra care.

o Your Role: Suggesting shared activities like yoga or light strength training can be a fun way to stay active together and support her health.

4. Hot Flashes and Night Sweats:

o What's Happening: Imagine her internal thermostat going haywire, causing sudden waves of heat. These aren't just uncomfortable—they can be downright disruptive.

o Your Role: Keep the house cool, invest in breathable sheets, and never complain about how cold the room feels.

Navigating Physical Challenges Together

These changes can feel like a betrayal to her body. Your job? Be her ally in adapting to this new normal. Here's how:

• Stay Active Together: Exercise isn't just great for physical health—it's also a mood booster. Make it fun! Dance in the living room, hike a local trail, or take a class together.

• Celebrate Small Wins: If she's proud of fitting into her jeans or sticking to her new routine, celebrate it! Positive reinforcement goes a long way.

• Keep Your Perspective: While she might feel self-conscious about changes, remember that she's still the same person you fell for. Don't just say it—show it.

Humor Meets Hormones

Let's face it: some of these changes can be funny when you look at them through the right lens.

• Hot Flash Humor: Imagine her jumping into the fridge and declaring it her new happy place.

• The Quest for Comfortable Clothes: She'll likely start favoring breathable fabrics and elastic waistbands. Your job is to admire her new "lounging chic" aesthetic without hesitation.

The Key is Compassion

The physical changes of menopause can be frustrating and even embarrassing for her. Approach this phase with humor, kindness, and understanding. She doesn't need you to "fix" anything—she just needs you to be her cheerleader, her comedian, and occasionally, her air conditioning technician.

4 THE PERI-MENOPAUSE SNEAK ATTACK

Before menopause officially rolls out the red carpet, peri-menopause—its stealthy little sister—sneaks in unannounced. This phase, which can start as early as her late 30s or 40s, is when her hormones begin their gradual descent into chaos. Peri-menopause is the "soft opening" to the main event, and chances are, she won't even realize it's happening at first.

What Is Peri-Menopause?

Peri-menopause (aka "around menopause") is the transitional phase leading up to menopause, marked by hormonal fluctuations that can last anywhere from a few months to over a decade. Yep, you read that right: a decade. This is when the first cracks in the hormonal dam start to appear, with symptoms that come and go unpredictably.

Think of it as the annoying commercial break before the big game—except this one involves mood swings, irregular periods, and nights spent sweating through the sheets.

The Symptoms: The Sneak Preview

Here's what you (and she) might notice:
1.   Irregular Periods: Her once-predictable cycle starts playing hopscotch. Some months it's there, some months it's not, and sometimes it's a surprise attack.
o   Your Job: Stock up on supplies without grumbling. Periods don't stop cold turkey—they just get unpredictable.

2.   Mood Swings: Emotional outbursts might make an early debut.

5 INTIMACY DURING MENOPAUSE – REKINDLING ROMANCE WHILE NAVIGATING CHANGE

Menopause doesn't just shake up her body and emotions—it can also impact your intimate life. The hormonal shifts happening in her body may bring challenges that require patience, communication, and creativity. But don't worry! This phase doesn't mean romance is off the table. In fact, with understanding and effort, it can deepen your connection in new and meaningful ways.

What's Changing in the Bedroom?
1.   Lower Libido:
o   What's Happening: With declining estrogen and testosterone levels, her interest in sex might fluctuate or diminish. It's not a reflection of you; it's her body responding to its new chemistry.

o   Your Role: Approach this with compassion, not pressure. A non-judgmental conversation about what she's feeling can open the door to understanding and new possibilities.

2.   Physical Discomfort:
o   What's Happening: Vaginal dryness and changes in elasticity are common during menopause, making intimacy less comfortable.

o   Your Role: Be proactive and supportive. Encourage her to explore solutions like lubricants or consult her doctor for advice.

3.   Emotional Barriers:
o   What's Happening: With mood swings, body image concerns, and fatigue, intimacy might feel like the last thing on her mind.

o   Your Role: Build her confidence through compliments and thoughtful gestures. Intimacy starts outside the bedroom—with kindness, humor, and emotional connection.

How to Keep the Spark Alive

1.   Redefine Intimacy:
Menopause is an opportunity to rethink what intimacy means. Holding hands, giving each other massages, or spending quality time together can be just as meaningful as physical intimacy.

2.   Communicate Openly:
Don't tiptoe around the topic. Ask her how she's feeling and share your feelings too. Approach the conversation with care, focusing on teamwork rather than frustration.

3.   Try New Things Together:
Whether it's a weekend getaway, a couples' dance class, or even experimenting in the kitchen, shared experiences can reignite connection and closeness.

4.   Be Patient:
There will be good days and not-so-good days. The key is to stay consistent in your support, showing her that you're in this together.

Lighten the Mood with Laughter
Menopause can make intimacy feel more like an obstacle course than a romantic evening. Instead of letting frustration take over, find the humor in the situation.

Example: If she pulls out a tube of lubricant with the enthusiasm of someone wielding a fire extinguisher, crack a joke: "Well, I guess we're ready for liftoff!" Laughter breaks the ice and helps you both relax.

Practical Tips for Rekindling Romance

- Create a Romantic Environment: A little effort can go a long way. Light candles, play music, and take time to focus on each other.

- Focus on Foreplay: Hormonal changes mean she may need more time to feel ready. Approach intimacy with patience and creativity.
- Explore Professional Help: If intimacy becomes a source of stress, consider seeing a therapist or doctor together to explore options.

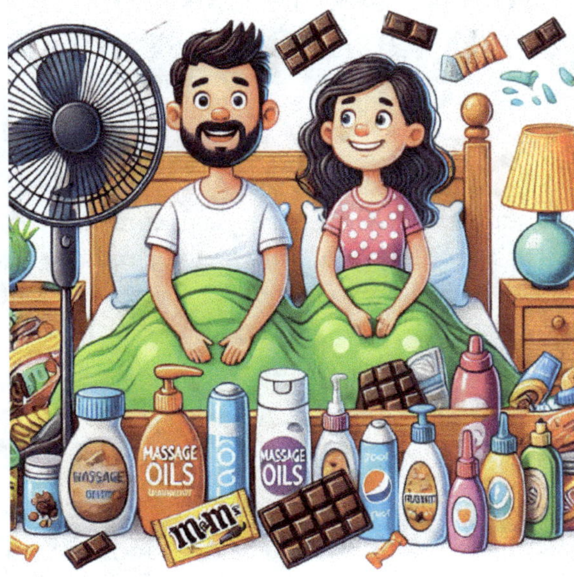

The goal during menopause is to adapt, not avoid. By embracing these changes as a team, you'll come out of this phase stronger, closer, and maybe even laughing more than ever before.

6 THE MENOPAUSE SURVIVAL TOOLKIT – GADGETS, PRODUCTS, AND MUST-HAVE TIPS

Menopause is no joke, but with the right tools, navigating it can be a lot easier—for her and for you. Think of this chapter as a survival guide, packed with practical suggestions to smooth the bumps, cool the heat, and lighten the load. Whether it's products, routines, or just clever hacks, these tools will help you both weather the storm with a smile.

Tools for Physical Comfort

1. Cooling Gadgets:
o Must-Have: Cooling pillows, portable fans, and moisture-wicking sleepwear.

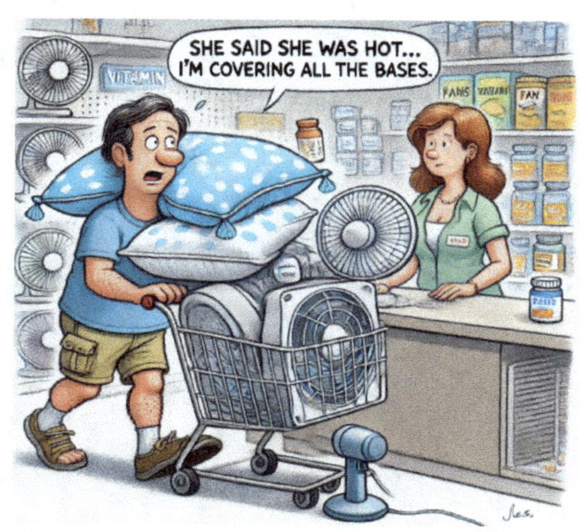

o Why: Hot flashes and night sweats can feel like sleeping on the sun. These gadgets are lifesavers for her—and keep you from waking up in a puddle of sweat.
o Pro Tip: A bedside fan with a remote control? Genius.

7 THE MENOPAUSE MYTHBUSTERS – DEBUNKING COMMON MISCONCEPTIONS ABOUT THIS JOURNEY

Menopause has been surrounded by myths, half-truths, and downright ridiculous assumptions for centuries. As her partner, it's important to separate fact from fiction so you can be a supportive, informed ally. Let's bust some of the most common menopause myths together—because misinformation doesn't help anyone.

Myth 1: Menopause Only Affects Women "Of a Certain Age"
• The Truth: While menopause typically occurs in the 40s or 50s, peri-menopause can start much earlier, sometimes in the late 30s.
• Why It Matters: If she starts experiencing symptoms sooner than expected, don't brush them off with "You're too young for that." Acknowledgment is key.

Myth 2: Menopause Means the End of Intimacy
• The Truth: Menopause may bring challenges to intimacy, but it doesn't mean romance or connection has to stop. Communication, creativity, and a little patience go a long way.
• Why It Matters: The belief that menopause marks the "end" can lead to unnecessary feelings of insecurity or distance. Embrace the opportunity to redefine intimacy together.

Myth 3: Hot Flashes Happen to Everyone

• The Truth: While hot flashes are common, not all women experience them. Symptoms vary widely, and what one woman goes through can be completely different for another.

• Why It Matters: Avoid making assumptions or jokes about her symptoms. Instead, ask her how she feels and what she's experiencing.

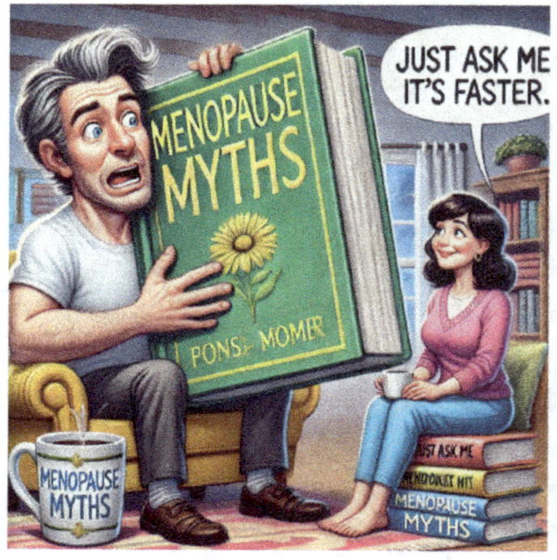

Myth 4: Mood Swings Mean She's Overreacting

• The Truth: Mood swings during menopause are caused by legitimate hormonal fluctuations, not overreaction or dramatics.

• Why It Matters: Dismissing her feelings will only cause frustration. Instead, offer empathy and a willingness to listen.

Myth 5: It's All About Estrogen

• The Truth: While estrogen levels do decline during menopause, other hormones—like progesterone and testosterone—also play a role. The body is experiencing a complex hormonal symphony (or cacophony).

• Why It Matters: Understanding that menopause is multifaceted will help you avoid oversimplifying her experience.

Myth 6: Once It's Over, Everything Goes Back to Normal

• The Truth: Post-menopause is a new phase of life, not a return to pre-menopause. Symptoms may taper off, but some changes—like reduced estrogen—are long-term.

• Why It Matters: Viewing menopause as a linear journey oversimplifies its complexity. Be prepared to adapt to ongoing shifts.

How to Be a Mythbuster

1.   Do Your Research:
Pick up books (like this one!), attend seminars, or read reliable online resources. The more you know, the better you'll be at supporting her.

2.   Ask, Don't Assume:
Menopause looks different for every woman. Ask her how she's feeling and let her be the expert on her own body.

3.   Challenge Stereotypes:
Whether it's a joke in a sitcom or advice from a buddy, don't let outdated notions cloud your perspective.

Empower Her (and Yourself) With the Truth

Busting these myths is about more than just avoiding mistakes—it's about fostering deeper understanding and connection. When you approach menopause with accurate knowledge and an open mind, you strengthen your relationship and show her that you're truly in her corner.

8 COMMUNICATION 101

When it comes to navigating menopause, communication isn't just important—it's essential. Think of it as the secret weapon in your survival kit. But here's the tricky part: menopause has a way of turning even the simplest conversations into a game of emotional Jenga. One wrong move, and the whole thing could collapse.

This chapter is all about giving you the tools to talk (and listen) like a pro, so you can be the supportive partner she needs without unintentionally lighting any emotional fuses.

Do's and Don'ts of Menopause Communication

Let's start with the basics: what to say and, more importantly, what not to say.

DO:
- Ask Open-Ended Questions:

Instead of guessing what she needs, ask: "How can I support you right now?" or "What would make today easier for you?"
- Validate Her Feelings:

Phrases like, "I can see how that would be frustrating" or "I'm here if you want to talk" go a long way. Even if you don't fully understand what she's feeling, showing empathy is key.
- Be Patient and Nonjudgmental:

If she needs to vent, let her. This isn't the time to jump in with solutions (we'll get to that later).

DON'T:
- Say, "Are You Sure It's Not in Your Head?"

Spoiler alert: It's not in her head—it's in her hormones. This phrase will only escalate things. Trust me.
- Play the Hormone Card:

While it might be tempting to blame her mood swings or irritability on menopause, pointing it out is like poking a bear. Just don't.
- Minimize Her Experience:

Saying things like, "It's not that bad" or "It's just a phase" invalidates what she's going through. Even if you think you're being reassuring, it won't land that way.

How to Survive Menopause Conversations Without Becoming the Bad Guy

Here's the thing: Menopause can make conversations feel like walking through a minefield. The key is learning to defuse tension before it escalates.

1. Master the Art of Active Listening:

When she talks, put your phone down, make eye contact, and nod occasionally. Repeat back what you hear to show you're paying attention:
- o   Her: "I feel so exhausted lately, and it's driving me crazy!"
- o   You: "You've been feeling really tired, and it's frustrating. I'm sorry—how can I help?"

2. Know When to Zip It:

Sometimes, she doesn't want advice—she just wants to be heard. If you're not sure what she needs, ask:
- "Do you want me to help figure this out, or do you just need me to listen?"

3. Use Humor Carefully:

A well-timed joke can lighten the mood, but the wrong one can backfire spectacularly. Rule of thumb: If you're not 100% sure it's funny, save it for later.

Proactive Communication Tips

The best way to avoid arguments? Get ahead of them. Here's how to be proactive in your conversations:

- Check In Regularly:

A simple "How are you feeling today?" can open the door to meaningful dialogue. It shows you care and keeps her from feeling isolated.

- Acknowledge the Elephant in the Room:

If menopause symptoms are affecting your relationship, don't sweep them under the rug. Approach the topic gently: "I've noticed you've been feeling a bit stressed lately. Is there anything I can do to help?"

- Set Boundaries (Respectfully):

If you're feeling overwhelmed, it's okay to take a step back—as long as you communicate it kindly. Example: "I want to be there for you, but I also need a little time to recharge. Let's figure this out together."

What to Say in Tough Situations

Sometimes, words fail you. Here's a cheat sheet for those tricky moments:

- When She's Having a Bad Day:
o "I'm sorry today's been rough. Let me take something off your plate."
- When She's Emotional:
o "I can see this is really hard for you. I'm here if you need me."
- When She Snaps at You:
o "I didn't mean to upset you. Let's talk about this when you're ready."
- When You Don't Know What to Say:
o "I don't know exactly what you're going through, but I'm here for you."

The Power of Non-Verbal Communication

Sometimes, actions speak louder than words. Here are a few non-verbal ways to show your support:

- Surprise Her: Bring her favorite snack or a cup of tea without being asked.
- Be Present: Sit with her, hold her hand, or just be nearby. Your presence alone can be comforting.
- Write a Note: A short, thoughtful note like "I'm so proud of how strong you are" can mean the world.

Final Words on Communication

Menopause isn't just a physical journey—it's an emotional one. The way you communicate during this time can strengthen your bond or, well, test it. By approaching conversations with empathy, humor, and patience, you'll show her that she's not in this alone. And that's what matters   most.

9 BE HER MVP
(MENOPAUSE VALUABLE PARTNER)

You've already started navigating the hormonal rollercoaster and emotional whiplash that menopause brings. Now, it's time to level up your game and become the Menopause Valuable Partner (MVP) she needs. This isn't about being perfect—it's about showing up, stepping up, and sometimes shutting up (more on that later). Your goal? To be her teammate, her support system, and occasionally her personal assistant when she can't even.

What Does Being an MVP Look Like?

Think of yourself as her partner-in-crime through this hormonal heist. It's not about grand gestures (though those are nice); it's about consistent, everyday support that makes her life easier and shows her you care.

Sharing Household Responsibilities

Menopause can drain her energy faster than you can say "hot flash." She might not have the stamina to keep up with her usual routines, and that's where you step in. Here's how to make it work:

1.   Divide and Conquer:
If you don't already share chores, now's the time to start. Whether it's cooking, cleaning, or tackling the never-ending laundry, taking on more of the load will give her much-needed breathing room.

2.   Anticipate Needs:
Don't wait for her to ask you to vacuum or take out the trash. Proactively look for ways to help—like noticing the dishes piling up or the dog giving you the "I need a walk" eyes.

3.   Offer, Don't Hover:
If she insists on handling certain tasks herself, let her. But offer to help without hovering like a helicopter partner. Say, "Let me know if you need a hand," and mean it.

Stocking Emergency Chocolate (and Other Essentials)

Menopause often brings intense cravings, and chocolate is practically a universal love language. But it's not just about snacks—it's about paying attention to her little comfort items. Build her a menopause survival kit stocked with:
- Chocolate (obviously).
- Her favorite teas or beverages.
- Cooling towels or a portable fan.
- Moisturizer for dry skin.
- A cozy blanket for when she's feeling chilly.

Pro Tip: Keep these items handy without making a big deal out of it. You're her MVP, not her supplier.

Practicing Patience Like a Zen Master

Menopause can test even the most serene of souls, but maintaining your calm is one of the best ways to support her. Here's how to channel your inner Zen:

1.   Pause Before Reacting:
If she snaps at you, take a deep breath before responding. Remind yourself that it's the hormones talking, not her. (Probably.)

2.   Repeat the MVP Mantra:
"This is temporary. She's worth it." Say it to yourself as often as needed.

3.   Find Your Own Outlet:
Supporting her doesn't mean ignoring your own stress. Whether it's going for a run, playing video games, or venting to a friend, find a healthy outlet to recharge.

Be Her Cheerleader, Not Her Fixer

When she's feeling overwhelmed, your instinct might be to swoop in with solutions. But often, she doesn't need you to fix anything—she just needs you to be there. Here's how to strike the balance:

•	Cheer Her On:

When she's having a tough day, remind her of how strong she is. Say things like, "I'm so impressed by how you're handling everything," or "You're doing amazing."

•	Support Without Smothering:

Offer practical help, but don't make her feel like she's incapable. For example:

o	Instead of: "You look exhausted. I'll do everything."

o	Say: "I've got dinner tonight. You go rest."

The MVP's Guide to Thermostat Wars

Menopause has a way of turning the thermostat into a battlefield. One moment she's roasting; the next, she's freezing. Here's how to survive:

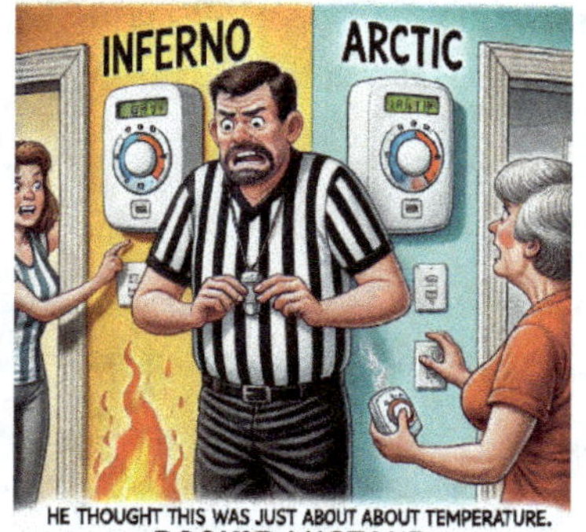

1.	Layers Are Your Friend:
Wear layers you can easily remove when she cranks up the heat—or piles on the blankets.

2.	Invest in Cooling Gadgets:
A bedside fan or cooling sheets can save your relationship (and your sleep).

3.	Don't Take It Personally:
When she's yelling about the "inferno" in the living room, remember: it's not about you. Just adjust the temperature and move on.

The Power of Small Gestures

Being an MVP doesn't mean overhauling your life; it's about thoughtful actions that show her you care. Try these:

•	Surprise her with her favorite coffee or a snack when she's having a rough day.

•	Write her a note that says, "You're amazing, even when you don't feel like it."

•	Plan a relaxing evening with her favorite movie, cozy socks, and zero interruptions.

Humor Is Your Secret Weapon

When in doubt, make her laugh. Menopause can feel heavy, and a little humor can lighten the mood. Example: If she's fanning herself with a magazine, offer to install a wind turbine in the bedroom.

Pro Tip: Keep the humor self-deprecating or lighthearted. Avoid jokes that might sound dismissive of her experience.

Final Words on Being Her MVP

Being her Menopause Valuable Partner isn't about perfection—it's about presence. Show her that you're in this together, through the hot flashes, mood swings, and midnight snack runs. Your efforts will remind her that even in the chaos, she has a teammate who's got her back.

10 THE HOT FLASH HANDBOOK

If menopause were a superhero movie, hot flashes would be the dramatic explosions that catch everyone's attention. They come out of nowhere, they're impossible to ignore, and they leave a path of destruction (usually involving kicked-off blankets and turned-up fans). In this chapter, you'll learn how to recognize, respond to, and survive the infamous hot flash, both as a bystander and as her MVP (Menopause Valuable Partner).

What Exactly Is a Hot Flash?

Think of a hot flash as your partner's internal thermostat staging a rebellion. Her body suddenly decides it's too hot and cranks the heat up to "volcano" for a few minutes. This can lead to:
- A sudden feeling of intense heat, often in the face, neck, and chest.
- Sweating (sometimes profusely).
- A flushed or red appearance.
- Rapid cooling afterward, leaving her chilled or drenched.

For her, it feels like being microwaved from the inside out. For you, it might look like she's in a sauna while the rest of the house is comfortably cool. Welcome to hot flash territory.

The Anatomy of a Hot Flash

Here's how it usually goes down:

1. The Warning Signs:

She might start fidgeting, loosening her collar, or grabbing at a fan. This is your cue: the flash is imminent.

2.   The Main Event:

Her face turns red, beads of sweat appear, and she starts muttering things like, "Why is it so HOT in here?!" Resist the urge to comment; just let her ride it out.

3.   The Aftermath:

As quickly as it began, it's over. She may be drenched, chilly, or simply irritated. Your job? Be ready with a fan, a towel, or a supportive smile.

What Triggers a Hot Flash?

While hot flashes can feel random, certain things might make them worse. Common triggers include:

•   Heat: Warm rooms, sunny days, or too many blankets. (Hint: She's probably going to hate that cozy fleece comforter you love.)

•   Stress: Tension can set off the internal fireworks, so keep things calm when possible.

•   Spicy Foods: If she used to love hot wings, she might start cursing them now.

•   Alcohol and Caffeine: These can aggravate her symptoms, so don't be surprised if her coffee or wine intake changes.

Pro Tip: Watch for patterns in her flashes and adjust your environment (and snacks) accordingly.

How to Respond to a Hot Flash Without Making It Worse

Hot flashes are uncomfortable, but the wrong reaction can make them downright unbearable—for both of you. Here's your game plan:

1.   Keep Your Cool (Literally):

If she's having a flash, don't complain about how cold the house is. Grab a blanket for yourself and quietly adjust to her comfort needs.

2.   Offer, Don't Overstep:

Say: "Want me to grab you some water or turn on the fan?"

Don't Say: "You're sweating like crazy—do you need a towel?" (This will not go over well.)

3.   Be Prepared:

Stock up on cooling tools like portable fans, cooling towels, and breathable bedding. The more you anticipate her needs, the less stressful flashes will feel for both of you.

4.   Stay Positive:
Humor can help, but tread carefully. A lighthearted comment like, "Looks like summer came early!" might work, but only if she's in a laughing mood. When in doubt, stay silent.

Hot Flash Emergency Kit

As her MVP, you'll want to be armed with the right tools. Here's what to keep on hand:
•   Portable Fans: Small, battery-operated fans are lifesavers. Keep one in your car, her purse, and on the nightstand.
•   Cooling Towels: These magic towels stay cool when wet and can help her cool down quickly.
•   Breathable Fabrics: Suggest lightweight, moisture-wicking clothing and breathable sheets to keep her comfortable.
•   Cold Water Bottle: Encourage her to stay hydrated and have cold water nearby at all times.
Pro Tip: Keep her favorite fan charged and ready. Nothing ruins a hot flash rescue like a dead battery.

How to Handle Hot Flashes at Night

Night sweats are hot flashes' obnoxious cousin. They strike while she's asleep, leaving her drenched and miserable. Here's how to help her (and yourself) sleep better:

1.   Cool the Bedroom:
Lower the thermostat, use a fan, and invest in cooling pillows and sheets.

2.   Layer the Bedding:
Swap heavy comforters for lightweight blankets she can kick off easily.

3.   Be Flexible:
If she needs to get up and change clothes in the middle of the night, don't grumble—just let her do her thing.

When to Laugh, When to Stay Serious
Hot flashes might sound funny, but they're no joke to her. Still, a

shared laugh can lighten the mood—if the timing is right. Here are some safe humor tips:
•   Laugh Together, Not At Her:
If she starts laughing about her "personal heat wave," join in. If she's not laughing, neither are you.
•   Make It About You:
Self-deprecating humor is always a safer bet. Example: "I think my ice cream melted just sitting next to you!"

Final Words on Hot Flashes
Hot flashes are one of the most common and disruptive symptoms of menopause, but with preparation and patience, you can help her manage them.

11 WHEN TO LAUGH, WHEN TO BE SERIOUS

Menopause is a journey filled with ups, downs, and plenty of WTF moments. One minute she's laughing uncontrollably at a joke, and the next, she's glaring at you for breathing too loudly. Humor can be a powerful tool during this time, but timing is everything. Use it wisely, and you'll lighten the mood and strengthen your bond. Misfire, and you might find yourself on the couch with the dog.

This chapter is all about navigating the delicate balance between laughter and empathy—so you can share joy without downplaying her experience.

The Golden Rule of Menopause Humor
Before we dive into examples, here's the golden rule: Always read the

room. Humor is most effective when she's open to it. If she's mid-hot flash or dealing with brain fog, now might not be the best time to crack a joke. Instead, aim for moments where she's already smiling or when the tension could use a little defusing.

When to Laugh

Laughter can be a relief valve in tense situations, especially during the wild ride of menopause. Here are some scenarios where humor might be welcome:

1.	The Ridiculous Situations:

If she's fanning herself with a pizza box because the AC isn't cutting it, this is prime comedy material. Lighten the moment with something like:

o	"Are we air-conditioning the pizza or the room?"
o	"Should I grab a fire extinguisher just in case?"

2.	Shared Experiences:

If you're both dealing with menopause-induced chaos, laugh at it together. For example, if she's waging war on the thermostat and you're bundled up in three sweaters, say:

- "At this rate, I'm going to need a parka and ski gloves."

3.	When She Starts the Joke:

If she's laughing about her forgetfulness or mood swings, join in! Let her take the lead, and add to the humor in a way that feels collaborative.

When to Be Serious

Some moments call for empathy and understanding, not jokes. Here's when to put your humor on hold:

1.	When She's Overwhelmed:

If she's venting about how tired, frustrated, or uncomfortable she feels, resist the urge to make light of the situation. Instead, validate her feelings:

- "I'm sorry you're going through this. It sounds really tough."

2.	When She's in Physical Discomfort:

A hot flash or night sweat isn't funny in the moment. Offer practical help instead of quips:

o   "Can I get you some water?"

o   "Let's turn on the fan."

3.   When She's Feeling Insecure:
Menopause can take a toll on her confidence, especially with changes in her body. This is not the time to make jokes about her appearance, energy levels, or mood. Instead, remind her how amazing she is:

o   "You're handling all of this with so much strength. I'm proud of you."

How to Defuse Tense Moments with Humor

Humor can be a lifesaver during those moments when emotions are running high. Here's how to do it without stepping on any landmines:

1.   Self-Deprecating Humor:
If she's frustrated about something, turning the focus on yourself can make her smile without invalidating her feelings. Example:

- If she's annoyed at the messy kitchen: "I'm so bad at cleaning, I think the dishes are judging me."

2.   Playful Solutions:
When she's grappling with symptoms, offer silly but harmless suggestions:

o   "What if we install a mini-fridge next to your side of the bed for midnight cool-downs?"

o   "Should I buy stock in fans at this point?"

3.   Acknowledging the Chaos:
Sometimes, just naming the absurdity of the situation can diffuse tension. Example:

o   If she's having a meltdown over a lost set of keys: "At least they're not in the fridge this time!"

Jokes to Avoid at All Costs

While humor can be a powerful ally, certain jokes are guaranteed to backfire. Avoid:

- Jokes About Hormones:

o   "Must be the hormones!" (Nope. Just don't.)

- Comparisons to Other Women:

o   "You're handling this better than my mom did!" (Yikes.)

-     Minimizing Her Experience:
o   "It's not that big of a deal." (Yes, it is.)

Pro Tip: If there's even a 1% chance your joke could come across as dismissive, skip it.

Building Connection Through Laughter

The key to using humor effectively is to focus on connection. Here's how to build moments of joy that bring you closer:

-     Inside Jokes:

Create little in-jokes that only the two of you share. For example, if her hot flashes have become a running theme, you might start referring to the fan as "The Heat Slayer."

-     Lighthearted Rituals:

Watch a funny movie or show together. Laughter is contagious and can help both of you decompress after a tough day.

-     Celebrate the Small Wins:

If she makes it through a tough week, toast to her resilience with her favorite drink and a silly joke: "Here's to conquering menopause one hot flash at a time!"

Here are a few real-life menopause moments that show just how funny things can get:

-     The Sleepwalking Blanket War:

One couple shared a story of how she kept kicking the blankets off the bed in the middle of the night, and he kept pulling them back on. It wasn't until she woke up freezing on the couch with a single sock on that they realized neither of them had been awake during the whole ordeal.

-     The Grocery Store Mistake:

A man accidentally bought decaf coffee instead of regular. When his wife discovered it, she made him return to the store and dramatically declared, "The fate of the world depends on caffeine!"

-     The Haircut Incident:

A woman decided to cut her bangs at 2 a.m. after a particularly stressful day. When her husband saw the results, he said, "I love it—it's so… avant-garde!"

Menopause isn't always funny, but finding moments of humor can make the journey easier for both of you. The trick is knowing when to laugh and when to simply listen. By staying attuned to her mood and balancing your humor with genuine empathy, you'll not only survive this phase—you'll come out of it stronger, closer, and with some pretty funny stories to tell.

Remember, your role isn't to fix the problem—it's to be her calm, supportive teammate. She'll appreciate your efforts, even if she's too busy fanning herself
to say it.

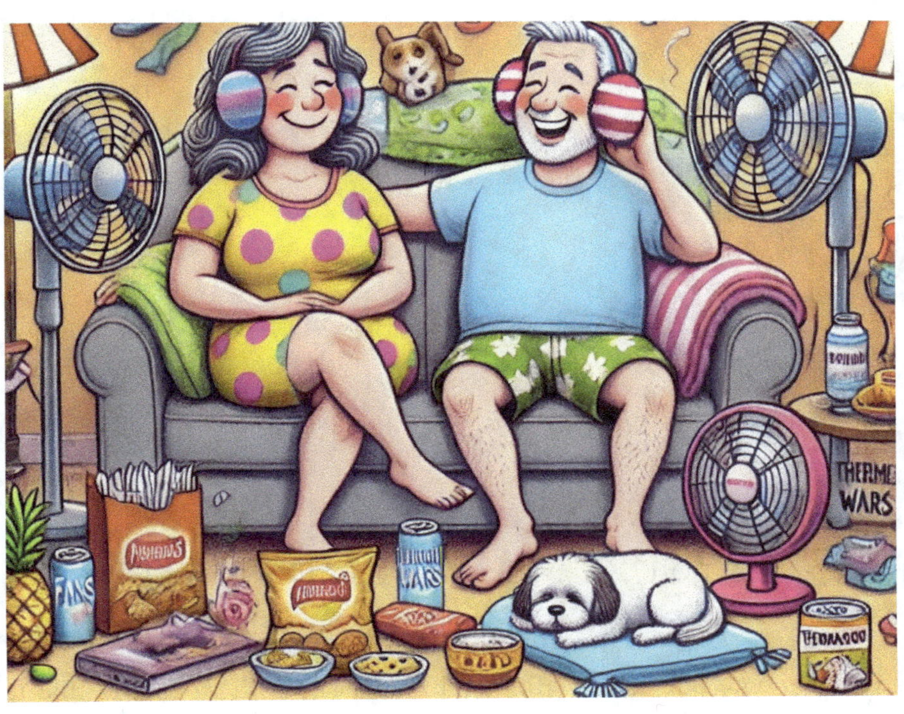

Agree to disagree, hold each other close (except when she's having a hot flash! Enjoy the moments, they all go to fast (except when she's having a hot flash)! Go with the flow (even when her flow stops following the schedule)! Expect the unexpected…tears, rage, laughter, appetite, craving, weight gain, frustration, energy, etc..

12 YOUR EMOTIONAL TOOLKIT

Menopause might feel like it's all about her—and to a large extent, it is. But here's the truth: supporting her doesn't mean neglecting yourself. If you don't take care of your own emotional health, you'll burn out faster than her thermostat during a hot flash. That's where your emotional toolkit comes in.
This chapter is all about giving you the strategies and support systems

you need to stay sane, centered, and supportive throughout this wild ride.

Why Your Emotional Health Matters

Menopause can be exhausting for both of you. As she deals with physical, emotional, and mental changes, you might feel like you're constantly walking on eggshells. The better you manage your stress, the more equipped you'll be to show up for her—and to keep your relationship strong.

The Essentials of Your Emotional Toolkit

1.　　Self-Awareness: Know Your Triggers

Everyone has limits, and understanding yours is crucial. If certain situations—like constant thermostat wars or late-night arguments—push your buttons, recognize those triggers and plan how to handle them calmly.

Pro Tip: When emotions run high, give yourself permission to step away briefly. Say, "I need a moment to process this so I can respond the right way."

2.　　Patience Is a Practice, Not a Virtue

Let's be honest: staying patient isn't easy when she's on her third mood swing of the morning. But patience is a skill you can cultivate over time.

o　　Take deep breaths.

o　　Remind yourself that her reactions aren't personal—they're hormonal.

o　　Focus on the bigger picture: this phase won't last forever.

3.　　Perspective: Pick Your Battles

Not every disagreement is worth engaging in. Does it really matter if she rearranged the kitchen again? Save your energy for the important stuff, and let the little things slide.

When to Step Back, When to Lean In

Being a supportive partner doesn't mean being a superhero. Sometimes, the best thing you can do is take a step back. Here's how to navigate that balance:

1.　　When to Step Back:

o　　If she's in the middle of a hot flash or emotional outburst, give her space to cool down—literally or figuratively.

o　　If you're feeling overwhelmed, it's okay to take a breather. Say:

☐   "I'm here for you, but I need a moment to collect my thoughts."
2.   When to Lean In:
o   If she's venting about her frustrations, be her sounding board.
o   If she's feeling insecure about her body or emotions, remind her of all the reasons you love her.

Building Your Own Support Network

You're not in this alone. Having your own outlets for support can make all the difference.
•   Talk to Friends:
Find someone who's been through a similar experience, whether it's a buddy, a mentor, or a family member. Venting to someone who "gets it" can help you process your feelings.
•   Consider Counseling:
If menopause is straining your relationship or mental health, couples or individual counseling can be a game-changer. It's not a sign of weakness—it's a step toward strength.
•   Join a Support Group:
Yes, there are support groups for men navigating menopause with their partners! They're a great way to share stories, swap advice, and laugh about the chaos.

Stress Relief Strategies for You

Managing your stress is just as important as supporting her. Here are a few ways to stay grounded:

1.   Exercise:
Whether it's a daily walk, a trip to the gym, or a few laps in the pool, physical activity can clear your head and boost your mood.

2.   Hobbies:
Don't lose sight of the things you enjoy. Whether it's woodworking, gaming, or gardening, make time for activities that recharge you.

3.   Mindfulness Practices:
Meditation, deep breathing, or even just five minutes of quiet reflection can help you reset during a tough day. Apps like Calm or Headspace are great tools.

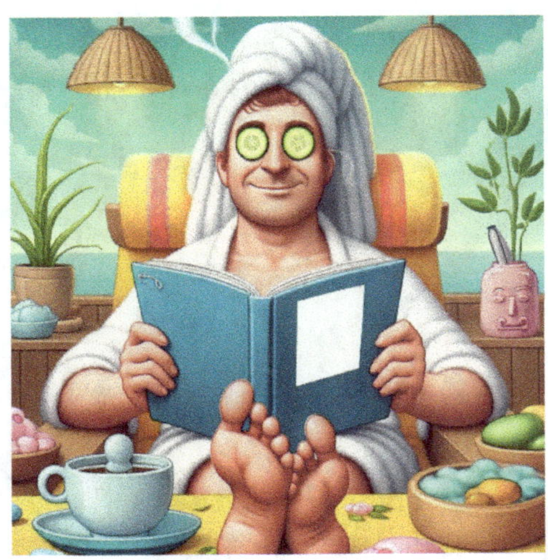

4.	Humor:
Find ways to laugh every day. Watch a comedy, follow a funny social media account, or share jokes with friends. Laughter is a powerful stress reliever.

Celebrating Small Victories

It's easy to focus on the challenges, but don't forget to celebrate the wins—no matter how small. Did you make it through dinner without a thermostat argument? Did she laugh at one of your jokes? Celebrate those moments.

Small victories add up, and they'll remind you both that you're in this together.

Final Words on Your Emotional Toolkit

Menopause is a marathon, not a sprint. Taking care of your own emotional health isn't selfish—it's essential. By managing your stress, finding outlets for support, and practicing patience, you'll be better equipped to navigate this journey together. Remember: you're not just surviving this phase—you're building a stronger, more resilient partnership.

13 UNDERSTANDING HER NEW NORMAL

Menopause is a life-altering transition, not just a phase. It brings changes that go far beyond hot flashes and mood swings. Her body, mind, and priorities are all evolving, and it's up to both of you to adapt. This chapter is about embracing her "new normal" with compassion, curiosity, and a willingness to grow together.

What's Changing, and Why?
Menopause isn't just about the physical symptoms. It's a time of reevaluation for many women, a natural point in life where she might reconsider her goals, values, and even her relationships. Here are some key shifts you might notice:

1.   Her Body Feels Different
Hormonal changes affect everything from her energy levels to how she feels about her appearance. Weight shifts, fatigue, and skin changes might leave her feeling less confident.
Your Role:
*   Offer compliments that go beyond her appearance. Say things like, "You're so strong," or "I love the way you light up a room."

2.   Her Priorities Might Shift
She might start focusing on new passions, relationships, or goals. Menopause often brings a desire to prioritize what truly matters and let go of what doesn't.
Your Role:
o   Support her exploration. If she wants to take up painting, start volunteering, or change careers, cheer her on.
3.   Her Energy Levels Are Unpredictable

Some days she'll feel unstoppable; other days, she'll need to rest. Menopause can leave her energy tank feeling a little unreliable.
Your Role:
o   Be flexible. Don't take it personally if she's too tired for plans. Instead, adapt and find ways to connect when she's feeling up to it.

How Her Needs Are Changing
Menopause brings new needs and boundaries. Understanding and respecting them is key to staying connected.

1.   She Needs More Rest
Sleep disruptions are common, and they can leave her feeling drained. Don't be surprised if she starts napping more often or goes to bed earlier.
Your Role:

- Create a restful environment. Turn down the volume, dim the lights, and give her space to recharge.

2.   She Needs to Feel Valued
Menopause can shake her confidence, especially with all the physical and emotional changes. She needs to know she's still the amazing woman you fell for.
Your Role:

- Remind her regularly how much you value her—not just for what she does, but for who she is.

3.   She Needs to Set Boundaries
As she focuses on her well-being, she might start saying "no" more often. This isn't about pushing you away—it's about making space for what she truly needs.
Your Role:
o   Respect her boundaries without taking them personally. If she needs alone time, let her have it.

Why She's Letting Go of Some Things (and Holding Tight to Others)
Menopause often inspires a "life audit." She might start letting go of relationships, habits, or commitments that no longer serve her. At the same time, she'll hold tighter to what brings her joy and meaning.
Your Role:

- Be her partner in this reevaluation. If she decides to quit a stressful job or drop a toxic friendship, support her decision.
- Help her nurture the things she loves—whether it's her hobbies, family, or time with you.

Rediscovering Your Connection

As her priorities shift, your relationship might need some recalibrating. The good news? This is an opportunity to grow even closer. Here's how:

1. Rekindle Old Traditions

Did you used to have a weekly date night or a shared hobby that's fallen by the wayside? Now's the time to bring it back.

- Example: Plan a picnic, take a class together, or revisit the place where you had your first date.

2. Create New Rituals

As her interests change, find new ways to bond. Maybe it's cooking dinner together, exploring a new hobby, or just taking a nightly walk.

3. Talk About the Future

Menopause is a natural time for reflection—and planning. Use this as an opportunity to dream together about what the next phase of your life will look like.

Adapting to the New Normal

Change can be challenging, but it's also a chance to deepen your relationship. Here are a few tips for adapting to her new normal:

1. Stay Curious:

Ask her about how she's feeling and what she needs. Show genuine interest in her journey.

2. Be Flexible:

Her needs and priorities might continue to evolve, and that's okay. Go with the flow and adapt as you go.

3. Celebrate the Changes:

Menopause isn't the end of anything—it's the beginning of a new chapter. Embrace this phase as an opportunity to grow together.

Final Words on Understanding Her New Normal

Menopause isn't just a physical transformation—it's an emotional and psychological one, too. By embracing her changing needs, priorities, and boundaries, you'll show her that you're not just her partner—you're her biggest supporter. This new normal is an opportunity to grow together, build deeper connections, and celebrate the amazing person she's becoming.

14 The "Pause" in Menopause
Why She's Suddenly Evaluating You, Her Life, and the Future

Menopause isn't just a hormonal rollercoaster—it's a life audit. It's as if the universe hands her a clipboard and says, "Time to evaluate your choices!" And guess what? You're on the list.

What's She Pausing to Consider?
Her Life:
Is she doing what she loves? Or is she just doing what needs to be done?
You might hear phrases like, "I've always wanted to learn pottery!" or "Why didn't I become a marine biologist?"

Her Partner (a.k.a. You):
She might ask, "Are we growing together, or just growing old together?"
Don't panic—this is your chance to shine.

Her Future:
This isn't about doom and gloom. It's about making the rest of her life the best of her life.

How to Support Her Without Becoming Her Audit Target

Encourage Her Dreams: If she says, "I want to backpack through Europe," respond with, "That sounds amazing! Should we pack snacks?"

Join the Journey: Help her rediscover her passions—and maybe even find some new ones to share together.

Be Patient: Remember, she's not questioning you—she's questioning everything. Stay supportive, and you'll both come out stronger.

15 Fueling the Fire (Not the Hot Flashes)

Best Foods for Menopause—and Recipes You Can Make Together

When it comes to menopause, food isn't just fuel—it's therapy. The right foods can cool the flames of a hot flash, soothe mood swings, and boost energy levels. Plus, cooking together can be a fun (and sometimes hilarious) bonding experience.

Top Foods for Menopause:
- Leafy Greens: Packed with calcium and magnesium for bone health and stress relief.
- Salmon: Omega-3s for mood and brain power.
- Berries: Full of antioxidants and sweet enough to satisfy cravings.
- Soy: Helps balance hormones (and it's a great excuse to order sushi).
- Dark Chocolate: Because…chocolate. Enough said.

3 Recipes for the Menopause Kitchen

1. Cool & Calm Smoothie

Ingredients: Spinach, frozen berries, half a banana, soy milk, chia seeds.
Directions: Blend until smooth. Serve with a smile and a straw.
Why It's Great: Fights inflammation, balances hormones, and tastes like dessert.

2. Omega-3 Salmon Wraps

Ingredients: Cooked salmon, whole-grain wraps, avocado slices, mixed greens, and a drizzle of lemon-tahini dressing.
Directions: Assemble and devour.
Why It's Great: Brain food that's light but satisfying.

3. Chocolate-Cherry Bliss Balls

Ingredients: Pitted dates, almonds, cocoa powder, dried cherries, and a dash of vanilla.
Directions: Blend in a food processor, roll into balls, and refrigerate.
Why It's Great: Satisfies chocolate cravings without the sugar crash.

16 The Pains of Menopause
And Holistic Ways to Kick Them to the Curb

Menopause doesn't just bring hot flashes—it also delivers physical aches, joint pains, and a body that suddenly feels like it's auditioning for a role in a pain-relief commercial. But fear not—there are holistic ways to ease the discomfort.

Common Menopausal Aches:
Joint Pain: Her knees creak, her back protests, and getting out of bed feels like an Olympic event.
Headaches: Hormonal shifts often bring pounding temples along for the ride.
Muscle Tension: Her body holds stress like it's competing for an award.

Holistic Relief Tips:
Yoga & Stretching:

Gentle yoga can ease aches and improve flexibility. Bonus: It's great for both of you.

Epsom Salt Baths:

Magnesium-rich Epsom salts soothe sore muscles and joints. Toss in some lavender oil for ultimate relaxation.

Anti-Inflammatory Teas:
Turmeric, ginger, or chamomile teas are calming and reduce inflammation.

Acupressure Mats:
These prickly wonders relieve tension and improve circulation. Just don't step on one barefoot!

Menopause Massage Night
Turn her aches into an opportunity for connection:

Set the mood with soft lighting and calming music.
Use a warming massage oil (bonus points if it smells like eucalyptus).
Focus on her neck, shoulders, and lower back—these are common tension spots.

Don't forget: Ask for feedback so you're helping, not hurting!

17 TURNING CHALLENGES INTO CONNECTION

Menopause might feel like a series of obstacles, but it also offers something invaluable: the chance to deepen your connection. Every hot flash, mood swing, and sleepless night is an opportunity to show up for each other, to practice empathy, and to build a relationship that's even stronger than before. This chapter is about transforming challenges into opportunities for growth, laughter, and love.

The Silver Lining of Menopause
While menopause is often seen as a difficult phase, it can also bring unexpected benefits:
•   Increased Communication:
Navigating the ups and downs requires open, honest communication, which can bring you closer.
•   Deeper Understanding:
Supporting her through this time helps you understand each other on a

understand what she's going through.

o   Empathetic Responses:

☐   "I can see this is really hard for you."

☐   "I'm here, no matter how tough things get."

3.   Celebrate Small Victories Together

Each day brings its own challenges and wins. Celebrate the small victories, like making it through a tough conversation without an argument or laughing together during a difficult moment.

o   Celebration Ideas:

☐   High-five each other after navigating a tough day.

☐   Share a treat or plan a special evening to mark the good moments.

Final Words on Turning Challenges Into Connection

Menopause might feel like an obstacle course, but it's also an opportunity. Each challenge you face together is a chance to grow closer, understand each other better, and build a stronger relationship. By approaching this journey as a team, using humor as a tool, and celebrating each other's strengths, you're not just surviving menopause—you're thriving through it.

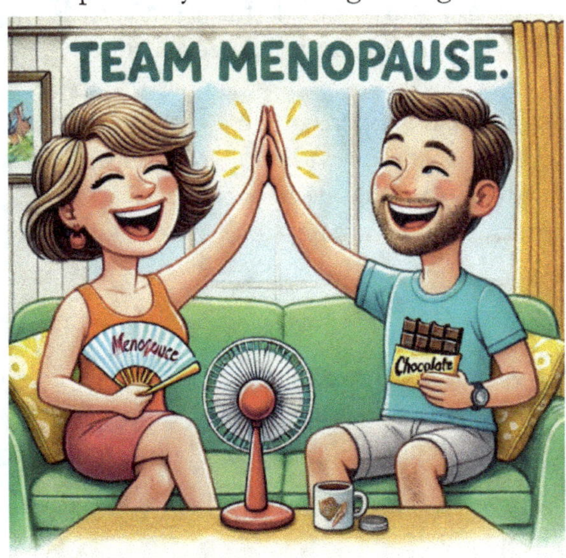

Coming up next: Conclusion: Why You'll Both Survive—and Thrive. Let's wrap up this journey with some final thoughts on navigating menopause as a team and coming out stronger on the other side.

Conclusion: Why You'll Both Survive—and Thrive

Congratulations! You've made it through the ups and downs of this guide—and hopefully, you're feeling a little more equipped to navigate menopause with your partner. Sure, it's been a journey full of hot flashes, mood swings, and midnight thermostat battles, but it's also a time for growth, understanding, and (believe it or not) connection.

Menopause isn't just something that happens to her—it's something that affects both of you. And by showing up with empathy, humor, and a willingness to adapt, you've proven that you're more than just a bystander. You're her partner, her teammate, and, yes, her MVP (Menopause Valuable Partner).

What You've Learned
Here's a quick recap of the tools and insights you've gained:
1.   Understanding the Hormonal Chaos:
You've learned the basics of what's happening in her body—and why her thermostat seems to have a mind of its own.

2.   How to Support Without Smothering:
You know when to step in, when to step back, and how to offer practical help without overstepping.

3.   The Power of Humor:
You've mastered the fine art of laughing with her (not at her) and using humor to defuse tension and lighten the mood.

4.   Taking Care of Yourself:
You've realized that your emotional and physical health matter, too—and that self-care isn't selfish; it's essential.

5.   Turning Challenges Into Connection:
You've discovered how to turn even the toughest moments into opportunities to grow closer as a couple.

Why You'll Both Survive—and Thrive
Menopause isn't the end of anything—it's the beginning of a new chapter. Yes, it comes with its challenges, but it's also a time for reflection, growth, and reinvention. By navigating this journey together, you're not just surviving—you're building a relationship that's stronger, more empathetic, and more connected than ever.

Encouragement for the Next Stage
The best part? Menopause doesn't last forever. While the journey might feel long, the lessons you're learning now will serve you both for years to come. Whether it's better communication, a deeper understanding of each other, or an arsenal of hilarious inside jokes, you're creating a foundation for the next phase of your relationship.

Here's what you can look forward to:
•   More Time for Each Other:
As life settles into a new normal, you'll find more opportunities to focus on your connection and shared interests.
•   A Stronger Partnership:
You've weathered this storm together, proving that you're an unstoppable team.
•   The Ability to Face Anything Together:
If you can handle menopause, you can handle anything.

Final Words of Wisdom

To the men reading this: thank you for stepping up, for caring enough to learn, and for being the kind of partner who's willing to tackle this journey with humor and heart. You're not just surviving menopause—you're thriving through it, and your relationship is better for it.

To the women: thank you for your patience, your resilience, and your willingness to let your partner be part of this journey. Menopause isn't easy, but your strength and grace make it clear why you're truly the MVP of this team.

Together, you've got this.

THE AUTHOR

Jennifer Erchul has been navigating the wild, unpredictable waters of menopause for 13 years with a sense of humor, a patient husband, three (mostly patient) kids, two dogs, and a cat named Keith Richards who seems to understand her mood swings better than most humans.

Jennifer's writing career began in 2002, well before blogging and content creation were mainstream. A pioneer of the "Work From Home" movement, she built a career crafting words for companies that needed blogs and an online presence but didn't yet know what SEO was. Since then, she's written for multiple industries and publications, always with a focus on making complex topics relatable (and, occasionally, hilarious).

While writing is her first love, Jennifer is a serial entrepreneur at heart. She thrives on launching new projects, bringing ideas to life, and finding creative ways to juggle chaos with caffeine. Menopause for Men is her latest endeavor, written to help men survive menopause with their sense of humor intact—and maybe even earn a few brownie points along the way.

When she's not writing, brainstorming her next big idea, or chasing Keith Richards off the counter, Jennifer can usually be found balancing life, family, and laughter in the hills of SE Idaho.

Extras: Appendices for "Menopause for Men"

Appendix 1: The Menopause Survival Kit Checklist

Your essential guide to keeping her (and you) comfortable, calm, and
the journey like a pro.

Cooling Essentials:
*   Portable fan (bonus points if it's rechargeable)
*   Cooling gel pillow or cooling pad for the bed
*   Moisture-wicking sleepwear and sheets
*   Ice packs (or her favorite frozen veggie bag for emergency cool downs)

Snacks & Comfort Food:
*   High-quality chocolate (don't skimp here—she'll know)
*   Herbal teas (chamomile, peppermint, or anything calming)
*   Healthy snacks like nuts, dried fruit, or trail mix
*   Her favorite indulgence (ice cream, cookies, or spicy chips—ask her!)

Self-Care Tools:
- Luxurious lotion or body oil for dry skin
- Calming essential oils (lavender or eucalyptus work wonders)
- A soft, cozy blanket for when the chills set in
- A favorite book, puzzle, or other relaxing activity

Emotional Support Items:
- Tissues for tears, happy or otherwise
- A journal and pen for venting or reflection
- Your undivided attention (free but priceless)

Your MVP Toolkit:
- Notebook for jotting down her preferences, triggers, and funny moments
- List of supportive phrases (see below)
- A sense of humor (pack this one every day)

Appendix 2: Resource Guide

When you need more information, support, or a good laugh, these resources have you covered.

Books:
• The Menopause Manifesto by Dr. Jen Gunter
A science-backed, empowering guide to understanding menopause.
• What Fresh Hell Is This? by Heather Corinna
A humorous and honest take on navigating menopause.
• Is It Hot in Here? Or Is It Me? by Barbara Kantrowitz and Pat
Wingert: A comprehensive guide to menopause for women and their
partners.

Websites & Online Communities:
• North American Menopause Society (NAMS):
www.menopause.org
Evidence-based information and resources for menopause support.
• Reddit: r/Menopause
A community of women (and some men) sharing real-life experiences
And advice.
• Hot Flash Havoc:
www.hotflashhavoc.net

Educational resources with a touch of humor.
Experts & Podcasts:
•   Menopause Matters Podcast: Hosted by Dr. Louise Newson, this
podcast dives into all things menopause with expert advice.
•   The Midlife Feast Podcast: A lighthearted look at nutrition and
Lifestyle changes during menopause.
•   Your Partner's Doctor: Encourage her to talk to her healthcare
provider about symptoms and options—this journey is unique for
every woman.

Appendix 3: Quick Reference Cheat Sheet Hormones in Play:

•   Estrogen: Declines during menopause, leading to hot flashes,
mood
swings, and changes in skin and energy levels.
•   Progesterone: The calming hormone that also drops, sometimes
increasing anxiety or irritability.
•   Testosterone: Declines too, affecting libido and energy.

Common Symptoms:

•   Hot flashes and night sweats
•   Mood swings and irritability

- Fatigue and brain fog
- Vaginal dryness and changes in libido
- Weight gain or redistribution (hello, midsection)
- Insomnia or sleep disruptions

What **NOT** to Say (Ever):

- "Is it really that bad?"
- "Are you sure this isn't in your head?"
- "Are you mad, or is it just your hormones?"
- "You're so emotional these days."
- "When is this going to be over?"

What **TO** Say Instead:

- "That sounds tough. How can I help?"
- "You're handling this so well—can I do anything to make it easier?"
- "I love you, no matter what."
- "Want me to grab your favorite chocolate/snack/tea?"

"The Menopause Waltz"
Oh, welcome, dear man, to the menopause dance,
Where logic is rare, and chaos takes a stance.
Her hormones are raging, her mood's a surprise,
One moment she's laughing, the next, teary eyes.

Her thermostat's broken—it's hot, then it's cold,
She can't regulate-she's ready to fold.
She's armed with a fan, and also a sweater,
She can't decide which one is better.

Chocolate's the answer, and snacks are the key,
To calm the wild beast of hormonal spree.
When she cries at a dog or a cute little cat,
Just nod and agree—don't question that.

She's questioning life, her job, even you,
Wondering if she needs something new.
Don't panic, don't run, just listen and say,
"I'm here, my love, through night and day."

Her joints may creak, her patience runs thin,
But her strength shines through from deep within.

Your job's not to fix, but simply to be,
A partner, a friend, her hot-flash referee.

So grab your guide, and embrace the ride,
With humor and snacks, you'll stand by her side.
Menopause isn't a war—it's a chance to unite,
To grow, to laugh, and hold on tight.

For when this storm passes, your bond will remain,
Stronger and closer, with love to sustain.
So here's to the dance, the waltz you both know,
Menopause for Men—let the humor flow!